I0791006

5 Best Ways To Lose Weight

When you are dealing with a phenomenon as diverse as human beings, it is very difficult to create rules which will work equally well for everyone. Nevertheless, there are some characteristics shared by all human beings, and this means that some basic principles can be developed. Here are five proven techniques to help you lose weight.

Best Way 1

The most fundamental strategy of successful weight loss is to burn more calories than you take in. You shouldn't find it difficult to apply this in some aspect of your life. Adjust your diet by cutting down on high fat food, and take some simple exercise for twenty minutes, three times a week. Going for a brisk walk instead of driving everywhere will have the desired effect, as will gentle jogging or swimming.

Best Way 2

Gym membership is becoming increasingly popular, and, as long the exercise you do is well planned, it can be extremely beneficial. Aerobic exercise has to be the focal point of your plan, otherwise you could do more harm than good. Provided you adhere to this basic rule, some anaerobic weight or resistance training can help tone up your body. This will give you more strength and vitality, and should increase your confidence.

Best Way 3

Going to see a professional nutritionist or dietician can pay off handsomely. If you go it alone, you will need to put in some serious research to make sure you are genuinely eating healthily, and many who try this find themselves discouraged by the lack of variety in their diet. It certainly doesn't have to be that way, as there are plenty of different healthy meals which help you lose weight. Getting the advice of a professional can make the task of losing weight seem so much more enjoyable!

Best Way 4

Find a friend to train with. If you and a friend are both regularly free at the same time of day, it can make sense to train together. Having someone to help you through the times when you don't seem to be getting anywhere can keep you in the game until the improvement suddenly appears. Having a social aspect to your exercise will help you look forward to it, and make you more likely to stick to it!

Best Way 5

Eat less food more often. Many medical practitioners now recommend eating more meals a day, with less food at each one. This is a more balanced way to take food into the body, spreading the load on the body over a far wider period of time. The system of eating three meals a day is designed far more to fit in with the working day than it is to fit in with the needs of the human body. When you eat less more often, the body absorbs more of the nutrients in the food, so your body craves fewer calories.

The best and most effective method for weight loss does depend on the individual, but follow these time tested principles and you will see results. Click the links below to discover some effective resources to help you.

Ephedrine and Its Use In Weight Loss

Ephedrine has been shown to increase the effectiveness of thermogenesis (fat burning) in the body. It contributes to the release and blocks the re-uptake of the neurotransmitter norepinephrine. This gives norepinephrine the ability to continuously stimulate receptors in your body, causing fat cell "flood gates" to open and facilitate fat loss resulting in weight loss. Not only does ephedrine increase the rate at which fat is lost, it preserves muscle at the same time, making it an ideal dieting aid for athletes. The most comprehensive look at ephedrine for weight loss is a recent meta-analysis published in The Journal of the American Medical Association. This meta-analysis was done by the request of the US Department of Health and Human Services. It reviewed 44 controlled trials on the use of ephedrine for weight loss it found that on average, it increased weight loss 1.3 lbs. per month more than placebo. However, combinations of ephedrine or ephedra with caffeine or herbs containing caffeine resulted in an average weight loss of 2.2 lbs. per month. Through nutrient repartitioning, ephedrine promotes fat loss while preserving fat-free mass.

One of the reasons why it is such a powerful weight loss agent is that it operates through a variety of mechanisms, including increasing levels of norepinephrine, epinephrine, and dopamine, and stimulating both alpha and beta adrenoreceptors. It (through facilitating the release of adrenaline and noradrenaline) stimulates the alpha(1)-adrenoreceptor subtype, which is known to induce hypophagia (appetite suppression). It is estimated that appetite supression accounts for 75-80% of the weight loss with ephedrine.

What is Ephedrine?

Ma Huang (Ephedrine) is known as one of the world's oldest medicines. Ma Huang (Ephedrine) is a member of the family of herbs known as the Ephedraceae. Ma Huang is a shrub-like plant found in desert regions throughout the world. It is distributed from northern China to Inner Mongolia. The dried green stems of the three Asian species (Ephedra sinica, Ephedra intermedia, Ephedra equisetina) are used medicinally. The North American species of ephedra, sometimes called Desert Tea or Mormon Tea, does not appear to contain the active ingredients of its Asian ephedra counterparts.

Ephedrine is a naturally occuring central nervous system stimulant obtained from the plant Ephedra equisetina. Ephedrine is produced by chemical synthesis, the synthetic product being marketed in the form of its salt, ephedrine sulfate; it occurs as a white crystalline powder with a bitter taste, soluble in water and very soluble in alcohol. Ephedrine's peripheral stimulant actions are similar to but less powerful than those of epinephrine (also called adrenaline), a hormone produced in the body by the adrenal glands.

What is Ephedrine used for?

Ephedrine has been used in China for more than 5,000 years to treat symptoms of asthma and upper respiratory infections. It has also been used in the treatment of headaches, fevers, colds, and hay fever. Today, compounds derived from this herb are commonly found in many over-the-counter (OTC) cold and allergy medications. Ma Huang is also found in some weight loss and energy products. For dieters, Ephedrine suppresses the appetite and stimulates metabolism through a process known as thermogenesis. Recently, Ma Huang has been the subject of scientific research for obesity because of this thermogenic fat-burning effect. It is used to increase heart rate, blood pressure and performance. This is normally released by your body under stress to enhance sports performance.

Ephedrine has moderately potent bronchial muscle relaxant properties, and therefore is used for symptomatic relief in milder cases of asthmatic attack; it is also used to reduce the risk of acute attacks in the treatment of chronic asthma. Ephedrine is also used to treat low blood pressure, because it constricts blood vessels and stimulates certain actions of the heart.

What are the side effects of use and Ephedrine Weight Loss?

Some of the more common side effects people experience from taking the drug are nervousness, dizziness, tremors, rapid heart rate, headaches, jitters, palpitations, insomnia, increased blood pressure. When taken at higher levels, ephedra can cause drastic increases in blood pressure, as well as cardiac arrhythmias. Discontine use if you experience any side effects.

Do not use this ephedrine weight loss product if you are now taking a prescription containing Monoamine Oxidase Inhibitor (MAOI) (Certain drugs for depression, psychiatric or emotional conditions, Parkinson's disease) or 2 weeks after stopping the MAOI drug. If you are uncertain whether your prescription drug contains an MAOI, consult a health professional before taking this product. Do not store above 30 degrees C (86 degrees F). Protect from moisture.

What is an ECA stack?

The ECA Stack is a component found in thermogenic weight loss pills, composed of ephedrine, caffeine and aspirin working to speed up the metabolism and thus cause calories to burn faster and result in weight loss. Anyone with high blood pressure or heart problems should not take the stack.

Benefits of Ephedrine (Ephedrine Weight Loss)

* ephedrine increases metabolism

* ephedrine suppresses appetite

* ephedrine preserves muscle tissue

* ephedrine treats symptoms of asthma and upper respiratory infections

Products And Programs That Can Help Lose Weight

Many available weight loss products and programs offer quick solutions to weight problems. It is a fact that it is a very hard task to achieve the desired weight. Before you get into a weight loss program, it is important that you check the cost of the whole session. Most of these programs offer high cost registration fees and may pressure you to buy pills and special supplements that will help you to have a physically fit body.

Over 50 million of Americans are engaged in weight loss programs, but only 5 percent sustain the weight they have worked off. Many people think that losing weight is easy; they may encounter the struggles of working out and dieting in the course of their weight loss programs. Many are still finding the most effective way to get rid of the excess weight in their body not realizing the fact that there is no such thing as a quick solution to get rid of the excess weight in a short time.

One solution that is seen by experts to be the answer to weight problems is the change of the lifestyle of a person. Eating healthier foods and having an active lifestyle only proves that it is the most effective way to lose weight.

Products that are sold over the counter to help you in your weight problems and even weight loss programs that enables you to have a regular exercise everyday can cost more money. If you want to engage in these kinds of programs, it is important that you must first get the enough information on how good the products or programs are that made others look good and achieve a physically ft body.

Although weight loss products and programs have the capability to help you lose the unwanted weight, it is important that you must select the program that can truly guide and help you in your quest for a physically fit body. To have a healthy diet could be the most recommendable thing that one must do to help the overall health aspects.

What You Should Know Before Taking Supplements

These days there is plenty of controversy and debate over whether it is beneficial to take various supplements. There are many kinds of supplements out there all with different intentions. There are food or meal supplements, weight loss supplements, strength enhancing supplements, and performance enhancing supplements, just to name a few.

While I do believe that certain supplements can provide some benefits for weight loss and increased fitness, taking the wrong ones or taking too high a dose can create some unwanted serious side effects. If you are either currently taking any supplements or are considering taking any then follow these tips to ensure they will not do you more harm than good.

For starters, get a physical checkup from your doctor. Talk to the doctor about what supplements you are taking or are looking to take and explain what you want to take them for whether it is for weight loss or to increase your strength for fitness. Your doctor can make sure that you have no conditions that would be adversely affected by them and may also have other recommendations as well.

Do your homework and learn as much as you can about the supplements you want to take. Many weight loss supplements for instance are only a meal replacement with a very high cost. You can start by using the internet to do searches on them. Here you can get plenty of information on them. You can also ask the local pharmacist, a qualified fitness trainer, or a qualified nutritionist about them for an even more in depth look at them.

Stay away from supplements that do not list all the ingredients or are a new, unusual, or unknown type. Stick with supplements that have a good brand name, use pharmaceutical grade ingredients, and make no lofty claims as to what their supplements will do for you like rapid weight loss for example.

When you do find a suitable supplement to take, never exceed the recommended dosage for any reason. No matter how good a supplement is, more is definitely not better. There is a very good reason why the manufacturer listed the dosage they did. Increasing that dosage with the belief that it will increase the effects of the supplement is the main reason people get sick or injured from using them.

If at any time you develop any side effects from the supplements you are taking, stop taking them immediately! The weight loss, strength, or general fitness boost you are trying to get from them is not worth compromising your health for. You may even want to consult with your doctor in case treatment is needed to ensure against further incident from the effects you may be having.

Many people take many different supplements every day for various reasons and some people do report positive results from them. There are supplements out there that are beneficial to take to help you with your weight loss and fitness goals, but just remember that there are a lot of bad ones too. If you are considering taking any supplements, follow these guidelines and more important, follow good common sense.

Tea: Drinking White Persian Melon Tea

White tea is fast becoming a very popular drink in the Western world. Once consumed only in China and Japan, and only for the most elegant of occasions, white tea is now being consumed as an everyday beverage for people all over the world.

White tea is special because of its very light and delicate flavor and fragrance. It's far milder and less astringent than black teas, and lacks the grassy flavor of many green teas. In addition, white tea has all the health benefits of green tea, and possibly even more benefits.

Like black and green tea, white tea comes from the camellia sinensis plant. But, white teas are harvested much earlier than other teas, before the leaves are fully open and while they retain fine white hair on the buds.

White tea is also processed differently than black and green teas, in that it receives the virtually no processing. The leaves are simply dried and steamed. The steaming prevents the leaves from oxidizing, protecting the delicate flavor and helping the tea leaves retain their natural anti-oxidants.

These potent anti-oxidants have been shown to slow down the aging process and prevent serious illnesses like cancer and heart disease.

The catechins in green and white tea have been shown to help speed up the metabolism and oxidize fat, promoting weight loss. In addition, white tea in particular seems to improve the immune system, helping your body fight off bacteria and viruses. Like other teas, white tea is high in fluoride, so it helps keep your teeth healthy, too.

One of the finest white teas available is a blend called white Persian melon tea. This tea blends the finest white tea with melon nectar for a refreshing and fruity taste. Not only does the addition of melon enhance the flavor of the white tea, but it enhances the health benefits, too. Melons are also a potent source of anti-oxidants.

Melons contain lycopene, vitamins A and C, beta carotene, and potassium. They also contain an anti-oxidant called GliSODdin, which has the power to eradicate some of the most destructive free radicals in the body.

In addition, GliSODin stimulates our bodies to produce its own anti-oxidants, and has been clinically proven to help maintain cellular health and protect against oxidative damage in several studies. These anti-oxidants produced by our bodies are far more powerful at neutralizing free radicals than the anti-oxidants we consume through diet.

So, now that I've convinced you that white Persian melon tea is a beverage you simply must add to your diet, you're probably wondering the best way to drink it.

First, it's important to begin with high quality loose tea. White tea is the rarest of all teas, which also means that it's the most expensive. However, even the finest white tea is affordable, costing less per cup than most sodas and gourmet coffees. Choose your tea from a reputable tea purveyor to ensure that you're getting only the best tea. White tea is less compact than other loose teas, so you will need more per cup than with many other loose teas.

Next, it's important to use fresh cold water anytime you brew tea. Put the water in a clean tea kettle and bring it to a boil on the stove. Put hot tap water in your teapot to warm it up while the water is heating. Once the water boils, remove the tap water from your pot and add your tea leaves. Use about 2 teaspoons per cup for white Persian melon tea. Let the water sit for a minute or two before pouring it over the tea leaves. This assures you that the water has cooled to between 170-185 F, the perfect temperature for brewing white teas.

Steep your white Persian melon tea for about 5-8 minutes, depending on your tastes. The tea will be pale with a golden color. Expect a sweet and fruity flavor with just a hint of smokiness. You should be able to get at least two infusions from high quality white Persian melon tea.

On those warm summer days, you'll find no better tea blends for iced tea than white Persian melon. The melon flavor, somewhere between the taste of honeydew and the taste of cantaloupe, is very reminiscent of summer and very refreshing. To make iced tea, simply brew several servings of tea at once and allow to cool.

Since white tea is so delicate in flavor, it's not wise to make white tea and then pour it over ice while hot. Doing so may dilute the flavor of the tea to a point that it tastes too weak. Instead, allow the pitcher of tea to cool before serving. This keeps the original flavor of the tea by not allowing the ice to dilute it too much.

You can also use your white Persian melon tea for cooking. In fact, one of the best ways to poach fish is in white tea rather than water.

Make about 2 cups of white Persian melon tea. Add other seasonings, such as lemon, salt and pepper as desired to the tea.

Sear the fish fillets slightly in a pan on top of the stove. When seared, add the seasoned white tea and allow the fish to cook until done. Try salmon, sea bass or tilapia with this recipe for a mild and delicious fish dish.

Experiment and you'll likely find many other ways to use white Persian melon tea, both for drinking and for cooking. You'll soon find out why this delicate white tea is one of the most highly prized in all the world.

The Magic Of The Thyroid Diet

Health & Fitness are considered most important in our daily life and our every day diet plays an important role in it. The Thyroid Diet has magical secrets of weight loss. Thyroid diet includes food you want to eat and lose weight overnight. Thyroid diet is the best for people who have weight challenges due to thyroid conditions. It helps us to return to a healthy weight, without a rigorous change in our diet and exercise.

The Thyroid Diet explores brands, mixtures and dosage of thyroid medicines right for us considering the other lifestyle issues and supplements that help to optimize thyroid treatment. It resolves nutritional deficiencies, treats depression and corrects brain chemistry imbalances, reduces stress, combats insulin resistance, treats food allergies and sensitivities, and exercise.

Thyroid diet recommends a very low-calorie diet for weight loss in cases of hypothyroidism but it is necessary to maintain metabolism. Low calories and lower metabolism sends body into hoard mode, which is a process, thyroid patients are susceptible to. Thyroid diet suggests breaking up calories into multiple "mini-meals" per day. The Thyroid Diet manages metabolism for Lasting Weight Loss. These thyroid conditions result in metabolic slowdown. The Thyroid Diet gives diagnosed and proper thyroid treatment for successfully loses weight.

This diet has many frustrating impediments for weight loss. It offers both conventional and alternative solution for help. The Thyroid Diet has optimal dietary changes. Thyroid sufferer have to focus on a low-glycemic, high-fiber, lower-calorie diet, optimal timing of meals for maximum hormonal impact, thyroid-damaging foods to avoid, helpful herbs and supplements. They face unexpected weight gain, despite diet and exercise showing symptoms as:

- Fatigue and exhaustion
- More hair loss than usual
- Moodiness
- Muscle and joint pains and aches

Hyperthyroid leads to metabolism that stores every calorie even after rigorous diet and exercise programs. Even optimal treatment doesn't help weight problems plague for many thyroid patients. For the majority of thyroid patients, treatment alone doesn't seem to resolve our weight problems. Thyroid diet is a simple, understandable way that offers you the support, encouragement and information to pursue the right diagnosis and treatment.

Safe Weight Loss Part 1.

Safe weight loss is about maintaining health whilst losing weight, it is not about losing weight rapidly; this has never worked and never will. This article is to be published in two parts over two days and will be stored in our news blogs archives for future viewing.

Aim for one pound (450 grams) each week because this level of weight loss is sustainable and you will not regain the weight later providing you adjust to your new healthier lifestyle.

Slow weight loss is the safest and most effective approach. A good weight-loss program helps you to lose weight gradually -- about one-half to one pound per week initially and improving to one pound each week. Gradual weight loss promotes long-term loss of body fat, not just water weight that can be quickly regained.

Diets are only half of the program because no program works without sufficient light exercise.

Most people leading moderately active lives need about 15 calories per pound to maintain their weight. For example, a 200-pound person would have to eat foods containing no more than 3,000 calories each day to maintain his or her weight.

To lose one pound, a person must burn 3,500 calories more than consumed. For example, reducing calories by 300 per day and increasing daily activity to burn off an additional 200 calories should result in a weight loss of one pound per week.

A Good Balance

When limiting calories, you still need to satisfy basic nutritional needs. Eat a variety of foods every day. Choose from each of the five food groups - dairy, meat, fruit, vegetables and breads - and allow for an occasional treat. Balanced food plans encourage making wise choices about everyday food; choices you can make to achieve and stay at your proper weight for life.

Evaluate Your Eating Pattern

You should also evaluate your eating patterns. Sometimes six small meals a day can help you control your hunger. If you prefer to stay with eating three main meals, always plan for some low-calorie between-meal snacks like an apple or a carrot to satisfy hunger between meals.

All foods and beverages can be consumed in moderation. Try to cut down on foods high in fat and sugar, or substitute with low calorie and low fat foods and beverages.

The choice is always yours.

Most successful weight-loss plans call for a reduction in both calories and the amount of fat eaten.

Exercise.

Determine what type of physical activity best suits your lifestyle. You should work your way up to regular aerobic exercise, such as brisk walking, jogging or swimming, since it is a key factor in achieving permanent weight loss and improving health.

Aerobic exercise works the body's large muscles, such as the heart, and should be moderately vigorous, but not exhausting, to be most effective. For maximum benefits, most health experts recommend exercising 30 minutes or more on most, preferably all, days of the week. I disagree with this because as you exercise and become fitter the amount of exercise that you do will become inadequate compared to your fitness level. My weight loss program recommends three sessions of ten minutes each week to start.

Try to incorporate some simple calorie-burners into your everyday routine. Even the most basic activities (such as taking an after-dinner walk, using the stairs at the mall instead of taking an escalator, or parking farther away so you have a longer walk) can get you prepared for more aerobic activities.

Part 2 of this article will follow.

This article is © copyright David McCarthy 2005. It may be reproduced only in its entirety with no changes or additions.

Weight Loss Diets - A Review Of 4 Popular Diets

There are a number of diets available, but here I review four which are popular at the moment.

1000 calorie diet

Trying the 1000 calorie diet is only advisable for one week, due to your body entering starvation mode and conserving fat. Overdoing the 1000 calorie diet is counterproductive to your body so try to stay on it for only 1 week. After 1 week you will loose between 3-5 pounds. The 1000 calorie diet can be used as a starter diet for a long term weight loss program. Try to aim for 2-3 pounds of weight loss and a good exercise program to begin with. After 1 week on the 1000 calorie diet, try upping your calorie intake or reverting back to a not so severe diet, this will prevent your body's metabolism from slowing down. Here is a simple 1000 calorie daily menu.

Breakfast

* Banana sandwich made with 2 slices of wholemeal bread and a small banana.

* Small glass of orange juice

Snack

* 1 pot of low fat yoghurt (preferably fruit)

Lunch

* 1 wholemeal roll filled with tuna and low fat mayonnaise (use tin tuna in spring water)

* Mixed lettuce salad, red or yellow sweet peppers, spring onions

Snack

* 1 bag of lower fat crisps

Dinner

* Roast chicken breast (without skin)

* Potatoes, mashed with 30ml semi-skimmed milk

* Broccoli (all vegetables steamed or boiled)

* Carrots

* Gravy (made from granules)

Evening

* 1 low calorie hot chocolate drink made with powder and water

Drinks throughout the day

* Diet coke, water, black coffee or tea without sugar

The 1000 calorie diet can be used as a starter diet for a long term weight loss program. Try to aim for 2-3 pounds of weight loss and a good exercise program to begin with. Remember after 1 week on the 1000 calorie diet, try upping your calorie intake or reverting back to a not so severe diet, this will prevent your body's metabolism from slowing down.

Vegetarian Diet

A well balanced vegetarian diet provides many benefits for the body. Some of those benefits include a reduced risk of chronic diseases, such as:

* Obesity

* Coronary artery disease

* Hypertension

* High blood pressure

* Diabetes

* Some types of cancer and more...

Your vegetarian diet, must be planned well. If not your body could end up in need of some vital nutrients. Some of these nutrients essential for the body are:

* Protein

* Minerals (zinc, calcium, iron)

* Vitamin b12

* Vitamin d

Protein sources include, tofu and other soy-based products, legumes, seeds, nuts, grains, and vegetables

Experts say that in order for a balanced vegetarian diet, you should eat nuts and whole grain cereals for good sources amino acids.

Greens such as spinach, kale and broccoli are a good source of calcium.

For sources of vitamin b12 which comes from animals, can be substituted with fortified breakfast cereals and fortified soy drinks.

Sources of iron are red meats, liver and egg yolks which are all high in cholesterol. Spinach, dried beans and dried fruits are all good vegetarian sources of iron.

A vegetarian diet is healthier than a meat diet. However this does not mean that you have the right to stuff your face with crisps, chocolate and chips everyday. Your balanced diet should include all of the above, i.e. Fruit, vegetables, nuts, dairy produce and soy.

Below is a table of some calorie controls in a vegetarian diet:

Food Group 1200 Calorie 1500 Calorie 1800 Calorie

Vegetables 5 servings 6 servings 8 servings

Fruits 3 servings 3 servings 5 servings

Grains 2 servings 3 servings 4 servings

Dairy 2 servings 2-3 servings 2-3 servings

Beans, Nuts and Seeds 5oz 6oz 7oz

Total Fat 30-35g 40-50g 50-60g

You can find a massive rage of diets on the internet free of charge! A vegetarian diet is an all round healthier option, and can go a long way to helping you on the road to losing weight.

Abs Diet

The Abs Diet works on the theory that every 1lb of muscle gained, your body intern burns an extra 50 calories per day. So if you can build an extra 10lb of muscle your body will then burn an extra 500 calories per day. Using the Abs Diet your body will burn more energy by eating the correct foods and exercising the correct way. Losing 500 calories per day will loose you 1lb of weight per week. Expect to loose up to 12lb in the first two weeks followed by 5-8lb in the forth coming two

The Abs Diet allows you to eat 6 meals per day which consist of 12 power foods, such as: chicken, turkey and other lean meat, olive oil, beans and pulses, almonds, low fat dairy products, green vegetables, oats, eggs, wholegrain bread, whole grain cereals, berries, and protein powder. All other food is a not allowed.

For 6 weeks you will eat a series of 12 power foods, which provide the body with all the fibre and minerals you need to stay healthy and build muscle. Along with the diet you will do a 20 min workout three times per week, which will aid in the fat burning.

The Abs diet is mainly aimed at men, however women are encouraged to participate. The range of foods you can eat is still good and you do get an exercise program out of it. Also some very good looking Abs, health and sex life. The full diet book is: The Abs Diet by David Zinczenko from all good on-line book stores.

The Kellogg's Cereal Diet

One of the simplest diets around at the moment is the Kellogg's Cereal Diet. It is not a crash weight loss diet which will loose you pounds upon pounds; however it will allow you to get into those jeans that are 1 size to small.

To start the Kellogg's Diet all you have to do is, eat one bowl of Kellogg's Special K or Cornflakes for breakfast, and also one for a replacement lunch or dinner. That's all! Carry this on for two weeks then you will see the results. Expect to loose around 3-6lb.

Whist on your diet, Kellogg's allow you to have the same drinks and snacks as you usually would, but recommend that you eat a well balanced meal every day, with more fruit and vegetables. Another tip from Kellogg's, is to keep a food diary to monitor and keep you aware of your current eating habits.

"Losing Weight? - Go Herbal"

These days, there is a great need for overweight Americans to lose those excess pounds. Being healthy would not only lead them to have a healthier lifestyle but it will also literally lighten their load, and improve their overall well-being.

There is a long list of dieting options available. There are exercise programs, exercise machines, dietary supplements, dietary food and drinks, diet pills - there are even soaps which claim to help you lose pounds while you bathe.

One other available option to shed off those unwanted pounds is to go herbal.

Herbal weight loss products have been in great demand for people who want to lose weight the natural way. However, when you take herbal supplements to lose weight, you would have to wait for a longer time for the results because of the more subtle effects of medicines which came from plants and natural herbs.

Here are some herbal weight loss options that you might want to consider:

1. Herbal weight loss products

There are a lot of herbal weight loss products available in the market now. You can check out the Internet and you will find a lot of herbal weight loss pills and products.

Be careful, however, as there are some products which claim to be safe and natural because they are herbal, but some actually have side effects because of non-extensive research on the effects of these products.

Here are some ingredients and chemicals which make up some herbal weight loss products that you should watch out for, as they might have harmful effects to your health:

> Senna. This is an herbal laxative. Senna is a main ingredient in weight loss teas, and it works by stimulation the colon. The downside effect of this herb is dehydration. It can also lead to colon problems and can become addictive. Some people, when addicted, are unable to perform bowel movements without it, so watch out.

> Chromium picolinate. This is a synthetic compound found in herbal weight loss products. Chromium is a nutrient which helps regulate blood-sugar level. However, this ingredient, when taken in high doses, may cause damage in the chromosomes. It can also lead to dehydration.

> St. John's wort. This supplement increases the production of a chemical in the brain. If not used properly, it may cause eye and skin sensitivity, mild gastrointestinal distress, fatigue and itching.

Although a lot of herbal products claim to be safe and natural, it is better to scrutinize the ingredients and research about the effects of the product itself before going for these herbal dietary pills.

2. Organic food.

In Wichita, Kansas, organic food has found its way to more homes and restaurants. Organic food devotees believe that consuming organic goodies help their bodies as well as the environment.

A person who buys organically raised eggs and vegetables claim to be healthier, and they are not spending money on doctors and prescriptions as these keep them healthier and away from the hospital. This could also be an option for weight watchers, as organic food is known to be kinder to your weight than chemically-processed food products.

3. Green Tea.

Studies show that intake of green tea, or green tea extracts burns extra calories. Also, green tea with caffeine can increase fat burning by up to 40% thereby reducing fat.

This is one good option for those who want to lose weight. In a study done, people who took green tea were found to lose 2 to 3 times more weight than those who did not drink green tea.

These results show that green tea is a natural product for the treatment of obesity. Thus, it also makes for a healthier dietary option, not to mention the good effects that it has on the body as compared to caffeine. A cup of tea gives an emmediate energy lift without the side effects of caffeine.

3. Caffeine.

Coffee provides an energy boost to increase fat burning. Caffeine also provides a likelihood to be active, which in turn increases your rate of calorie burn.

4. Immortality Herb

This herb, whose scientific name is Gymnostemna Pentaphyllum, is known to have the following benefits:

> increases healthy blood flow

> reduces artery blocks

> aids healthy blood pressure

> increases the rate of fat burning

5. Apple Cider Vinegar

There are pills and food supplements whose main ingredient is apple cider vinegar. Here are the benefits of taking this herbal option:

> weight loss

> improved cholesterol level

> improved high blood pressure

> helps prevent rheumatoid arthritis

A Guide To Positive Imaging For Weight Loss

Have you ever imagined how visualization can play an important part in losing weight and maintaining a healthy lifestyle that keeps it off.

Losing weight can be difficult for many people who use fad diets and pills to achieve their weight loss goals without letting their mind help in the process.

Visualization is a powerful technique that can help you make lasting lifestyle changes. Just by "day dreaming", you can significantly improve your chances in achieving your goals.

Visualization is a great weight loss tool and its as simple as visualizing your body as you want your body to look like.

This mental image of yourself is then transferred to your subconscious mind, which in turn starts to work on your body, shaping it in accordance with your mental image thus reducing your weight.

This means that if you program your subconscious with a mental image of yourself as a slimmer person, through persistence your mind will accept this and aid your body to conform to this mental image.

Once your mind is programmed with the proper mental images, it will start to work in assisting you to losing weight. I can't stress enough how important it is for you to believe in your visualization goals.

You have to let go of past dieting failures and refuse to entertain any negative images that come into your mind.

If you can visualize your body at its perfect weight and proportions, the subconscious mind will work to make it become a reality. It will then begin to positively reinforce your body into aiding the metabolism and eating habits.

Programming your mind into believing that you can lose weight, and to visualize yourself at your ideal weight is of the greatest importance.

Try to think of a different image of yourself, then let your subconscious do the work for you. If you think of your own body fat and being out of shape all the time, then the subconscious mind will find ways to make it so.

The subconscious looks after all of all your vital functions, it is the cause of all your good and bad habits, and also regulates muscle (the muscles are controlled by the subconscious) and body-fat composition on the body, and the latter is the one we are most interested in.

So please try to visualize your body as lean as you would like, and your mind will work on that image. The mind can be a great partner in losing weight.

Getting Rid of Bad Nutritional Habits

A bad habit is like second nature and is acquired over a long period of time. Bad habits are programmed into the subconscious and "will power" alone will not get rid of it. Many try using all sorts of different ways to break it but without success.

Obesity is the result of bad nutritional habits and some of the causes are boredom, stress, tension and different complexes. Food becomes the substitution for these causes and before too long, obesity sets in. Most people become concerned that they're obese, eat more and a vicious cycle is established.

The only way for lasting permanent weight loss is to break these bad habits and replace them with positive new ones, and the only way to do this is with visualization. Visualization puts you in charge of your subconscious where all these bad programs are stored.

All the will power in the world is not going to break these bad habits unless one has the help of their subconscious.

Relaxation

Relaxation the best way to reach the sub-conscious and will slow down the mind, turn off the exterior world so as to tune in to one's inner self. The best times for these sessions are in the morning and late at night right, just before going to sleep.

Try performing two sessions, one in the afternoon (primary) and the other before going to sleep (secondary) but once a day is quite sufficient. Sessions usually last 20 minutes, which isn't time consuming especially when taking in the benefits received.

When you begin your relaxation sessions, make sure you won't be disturbed - lock the door, take the phone off the hook and loosen all clothing. Now find a comfortable position, whether it is lying down or sitting in a comfortable chair.

Sitting may be preferable as you may fall asleep if you become too comfortable. You want to be conscious and not asleep in order to tap into your sub-conscious mind.

Try to exhale all the air from your lungs completely and then breathing in through the nose. Take ten seconds to fill the lungs with air (not to capacity, but comfortable) hold for ten seconds and then exhale slowly through the nose for another ten seconds.

Each one of these breathing cycles should last for 30 seconds, complete five cycles and after each cycle you will be feeling more and more relaxed.

If you are sitting, open your eyes and look straight ahead. If you are lying down, open your eyes and stare at the ceiling. After a few minutes, slowly close your eyes.

Having reaching this calm relaxed state start your visualizations. Put together images that power your emotions. Make them alive and colourful. Make the scenes as real as possible and imagine yourself as slim and toned the way you will look after successful weight loss.

Picture yourself ten weeks from now on the beach, walking briskly and confidently to your favourite spot, your breathing is normal and relaxed. You smile to yourself; you could keep walking like this for miles without feeling fatigued.

You lay your towel out and begin to take your clothes off revealing a firm, toned, well conditioned body. You have just bought a brand new swimming suit which just weeks before would have been lying in your closet waiting to be used.

Glancing around you notice the beach is busy, you catch the eye of someone of the opposite sex, they smile at you and you smile back. You walk confidently to the water and swim a couple of hundred yards with no problem or fatigue.

Or try this:

Visualize your family and friends complimenting you about how good your body looks and how slim you look. Try to view the scene as it is happening this instant - in the present, not in the future.

Using these visualizations you can construct in your mind any scene that desire. See yourself exercising, socializing, in the company of friends. Try and hear people complimenting you about your slim new body, and watch their admiring glances. Make the mental image as real as possible.

Remember set a goal for your ideal weight

You must want to lose weight

Visualize yourself at your ideal weight

Use positive images at every opportunity

Now that you are armed with this information practice these sessions on a daily basis and over a period of ten weeks you'll be on your way to become a happier and leaner person.

Tips on Minimizing Caffeine in Green Tea

When someone mentions green tea, what comes in your mind? Antioxidants? Health benefits? Weight loss? Caffeine? There are a lot of benefits that can be taken from green tea. Although, caffeine is not really ideal for most green tea drinkers. They may have some objections or second thoughts when it comes to drinking tea because of insomnia that can be caused by green tea's high caffeine content.

Worry not dear drinkers and advocates of green tea. There is a better way of drinking green tea without experiencing the effects of caffeine or otherwise minimizing it.

Tip # 1 - Start moderately

Fact is, a cup of green tea contains a caffeine level of about 20-70 milligrams. With this kind of caffeine in your diet, it's assured to keep you awake from dusk till dawn if your body is not used to drinking such dosage. Best advise is to take in small doses and try to observe your reactions. Start with a cup a day, then, when things still feel normal, increase gradually. Every time you increase, always observe for adjustments in your body. If you feel uneasy and somewhat irritated, then you can decrease to the level that your body can tolerate. If you are including it in your meal, and you're feeling more calm and contented, green tea is for you.

Tip # 2 - Get to know your tea

There are several kinds of green tea, Different kinds mean different levels of caffeine. It is stated by researchers that, the type of tea leaf used, the more caffeine it can produce. You can't indicate caffeine levels through color. Gyokuro is highly caffeinated compared to Lapsang Souchong which is a kind of dark tea.

Tip # 3 - Brew half strength

Very good solution for caffeine intolerance. To control your intake of green tea, you can choose to purchase loose green tea to allow you to adjust the way your green tea is brewed. The normal loose green tea brewing is at least two teaspoons. You can cut off the dosage in half. If you find the effects weak, increase it bit by bit.

Tip # 4 - Drink it while it's hot

Cathechin, the one that contains powerful antioxidants and theanine, this provides freshness and sweetness, can both decrease the level of caffeine activity of in the body. Brewing allows the molecules of catechin and theanine to combine together with caffeine in hot temperature. This will render caffeine to be less effective. If you let your hot green tea to cool off after brewing, the molecules that is bonded with caffeine will breakdown and releasing caffeine.

Tip # 5 - Avoid teabags

Compared to loose green tea leaves, green tea bags can't give you enough nutrition thus, giving you more caffeine in the process. Quality suffers from teabags. Rather choose green tea leaves that are loose.

Tip # 6 - Be familiar with your tolerance level

Several experts would recommend the consumption of not more than 300 milligrams of caffeine daily. Green tea has been found out that it can provide a steady and gentle source of stimulation. Side-effects like headaches and nervousness may be felt.

With these tips on how to minimize the effects of caffeine contents in your green tea, you can enjoy more tea with less caffeine.

www.ingramcontent.com/pod-product-compliance
Lightning Source LLC
Chambersburg PA
CBHW051141250726
48655CB00007B/3180